Crushing It with Keto!

Intermittent Fasting Blueprint

to

Thrive After 50

Alan Grodecki

Where These Concepts Come From

The principles presented in this book are not novel, experimental, or derived from internet trends. They are grounded in decades of metabolic research and the practical clinical work conducted by physicians and researchers who specialize in insulin, inflammation, fasting, and aging.

Medical professionals and scientists such as Dr. Jason Fung, Dr. Ben Bikman, Dr. Robert Lustig, Dr. Stephen Phinney, and Dr. Valter Longo, among many others in the field of metabolic health, have contributed to the mainstream acceptance of these concepts through research, clinical practice, and long-term patient outcomes.

Although this book is written in accessible language and draws from personal experience, the underlying concepts of lowering insulin levels, reducing inflammation, enabling the body to access stored fat, and utilizing fasting as a metabolic reset are well-supported by contemporary metabolic science.

It is important to note that this book does not constitute medical advice and does not advocate for the strict adherence to any doctor or protocol. Instead, it emphasizes the importance of understanding the workings of the body and employing proven principles to support its optimal functioning.

Table of Contents

Foreword: Your Comeback Starts Now

You didn't pick up this book because everything in your life was going smoothly. You picked it up because something inside you whispered – or maybe shouted – that it's time for a change. Maybe your knees are complaining more than usual. Maybe your energy fades before lunchtime. Maybe your favorite jeans now qualify as "aspirational wear." Or maybe you're simply tired of feeling tired.

Whatever brought you here, you're in the right place. And you're not alone.

This is the guide I wish someone had handed me years ago – simple, clear, doable, and built for adults over 50 (including those in their 60s, 70s, 80s…) who want to feel better without giving up their joy or struggling with insane exercise routines.

Keto combined with Intermittent Fasting is the most powerful, inflammation lowering, energy boosting, appetite calming approach I've ever used. And the best part? It isn't extreme, complicated, or punishing.

Let's begin crushing it together.

Chapter 1:
How I Stopped Fighting My Body and Finally Started Working with It

Turns out my body wasn't the enemy — it was just waiting for better instructions.

For a long time, I felt like my body and I were no longer on the same team.

Nothing was dramatically wrong—but nothing felt right either. The scale kept creeping up. My joints complained more than they used to. Mornings felt heavier, slower, and less forgiving. I was tired in a way sleep didn't fix and frustrated in a way no diet ever seemed to solve.

I kept telling myself this was just part of getting older. That feeling "off" was normal. That struggling with weight, energy, and health was just the price of admission after a certain age.

But deep down, I knew something wasn't adding up.

I had done what I was told. I followed the rules. Ate the "right" foods. Tried harder when things didn't work. And yet my body seemed to push back no matter what I did. The more I forced it, the worse I felt—physically and mentally.

There was no big breakdown or dramatic moment that changed everything. Just a quiet morning where I caught my reflection and thought, this can't be how the rest of my life feels. Not angry. Not desperate. Just honest.

That's when I stopped looking for another diet and started asking a different question: What if my body isn't broken? What if it's just overwhelmed?

That question led me to intermittent fasting.

At first, it sounded too simple to matter. Eating less often? Giving my body a break? That couldn't possibly make a real difference—especially after everything I'd already tried.

But something happened when I stopped constantly eating and started letting my body rest.

- The constant hunger faded.
- The mental fog lifted.
- Inflammation eased.
- Energy returned—slowly at first, then steadily.

For the first time in years, my body felt like it was working with me instead of against me.

The weight began to come off—not through punishment or obsession, but as a side effect of restoring balance. My health markers improved. My joints felt better. My confidence came back. And maybe most importantly, I felt capable again.

In six months, I lost 84 pounds. My diabetes reversed. My liver healed. But the real change went deeper than numbers on a chart.

I stopped feeling stuck.

I turned 60 feeling stronger, clearer, and more in control than I had when I turned 50. Not because I chased perfection—but because I finally gave my body the space it needed to do what it was designed to do.

That's why this book exists.

Not to overwhelm you. Not to demand willpower. And definitely not to promise miracles. This is about showing you how intermittent fasting can fit into real life—your life—in a way that feels sustainable, respectful, and empowering.

- If you're tired of fighting your body…
- If you feel like your energy, health, or confidence slipped away quietly…
- If you're ready for something that works with you instead of against you…

This book is for you.

And no matter where you're starting from, it's not too late to feel better again.

Chapter 2:
What Are We Really Crushing?

Right now, you might be wondering, "When do I eat? When do I fast?" Don't worry – we're getting there. But first, we need to get crystal clear on what exactly, we are crushing.

Spoiler: it isn't willpower, carbs, cravings, or even body fat.

The "it" you're going to crush is... INSULIN.

Insulin is the master and gatekeeper to your stored body fat – and one of the root causes behind stubborn weight, inflammation, metabolic slowdown, and a laundry list of health issues.

Every time you eat, insulin rises. Every snack, every sip of something sweet, every "healthy whole grain" moment – insulin jumps in.

And here's the real problem:

If insulin is elevated, your body cannot burn fat.

If insulin is elevated, your body cannot burn fat.

I wrote it twice because I cannot overstate its importance. This isn't my opinion – it's a well-established metabolic principle observed repeatedly in clinical and research settings.

You don't get to decide - Insulin decides whether your body:

- stores more fat, or
- releases fat for fuel.

When insulin stays high all day (like it does when we graze, snack, or follow old-school "six meals a day" advice), your fat stays locked away like treasure in a bank vault.

This is where Intermittent Fasting and Keto step in.

Both approaches keep insulin lower for longer, giving your body the time it needs to:

- access stored fat
- produce ketones
- reduce inflammation
- stabilize hunger
- improve energy
- support longevity

Why Lowering Insulin Changes Everything

When insulin stays elevated, your body stays locked in storage mode.

When insulin drops – through food choices and timing between meals (intermittent fasting) – your body finally gains access to its stored energy.

That shift explains why keto and intermittent fasting work so well together.

The detailed mechanics of ketosis, ketones, and cellular repair deserve a clear, focused explanation – and you'll get that in Chapter 6.

For now, remember this simple truth:

Lower insulin creates the conditions for healing, fat loss, and steady energy.

Why Old Diet Advice Failed You

You were told:

- "Eat low fat."
- "Eat every 2–3 hours."
- "Whole grains are heart healthy."
- "Snacking boosts metabolism."

But every carb-heavy or frequent bite triggered an insulin spike. Every spike stalled fat loss. Every stall increased frustration.

It wasn't your discipline that failed — it was the advice.

Even Drinks Count

Sugary drinks obviously spike insulin, but here's the curveball: Even some zero calorie sweetened drinks can trigger an insulin response.

This is why fasting windows work best with:

- water
- unsweetened tea
- black coffee

Give your body some space between meals, and it will reward you.

Our Simple Goal Going Forward

Lower the *frequency* and *duration* of insulin spikes. That's it.

And as someone who just turned 60, I can tell you – controlling insulin is the primary reason my quality of life and long-term health have significantly improved.

You're not just crushing keto and you're not just crushing fasting. You're crushing insulin – and claiming your health back in the process.

Chapter 3:
When Your Metabolism Starts Acting Its Age

At some point after 50, your metabolism updates its software without warning. Suddenly, foods you've eaten for decades start sticking to you like emotional baggage from an awkward family reunion. A simple weekend indulgence now requires a two-week recovery plan. And your body begins offering strong opinions about things it never cared about before — like bread, sleep, stress, and whether standing up too fast was necessary.

Hormones shift. Muscle decreases. Inflammation increases. Recovery slows. Your metabolism behaves less like a well-oiled, fuel burning machine and behaves more like a rowdy teenager.

Enter Janet, 57

Every morning, Janet followed the same routine: coffee, breakfast, shower, jeans. But one morning, her jeans fought back. Not a gentle nudge — a full rebellion.

She stared down at them. "We've survived holidays together," she muttered. "Why today?"

Nothing dramatic had changed. Her metabolism simply started "acting its age."

Why weight loss gets weird as we get older

- **Insulin** pushes your body to store fat.
- **Leptin** forgets how to signal fullness.
- **Ghrelin** (your hunger gremlin) becomes loud.
- **Cortisol** spikes from stress or poor sleep.

- **Muscle** quietly slips away.

None of this is your fault – it's just biology.

The good news

Your metabolism isn't broken. It just needs a different kind of support – the kind keto and intermittent fasting provide naturally.

This is where intermittent fasting shines.

By giving your body predictable periods without food, you lower insulin, calm the hunger hormones, reduce inflammation, and allow your metabolism to do what it's still very capable of doing – burning stored fuel.

Paired with a supportive low-carb (keto) approach, intermittent fasting works with your changing biology instead of fighting it.

- No extremes.
- No punishment.
- Just smarter timing.

And for people like Janet – and maybe you – that's when the jeans finally stop fighting back.

Chapter 4:
Inflammation: The Troublemaker Living Rent-Free in Your Body

Inflammation is like that roommate who never pays rent, eats your food, leaves messes everywhere, and refuses to move out. Modern metabolic research consistently shows that chronic, low-grade inflammation plays a central role in joint pain, fatigue, weight gain, and many age-related conditions.

You can't see it, but you feel it — in your joints, digestion, sleep, mood, cravings, and especially your weight.

Mark, 63, knew this all too well

One morning, Mark swung his legs out of bed, and it felt like someone replaced his joints with rusty hinges. He walked to the bathroom stiffly - like the Tin Man looking for a can of oil.

He wasn't lazy. He wasn't "out of shape." He was <u>inflamed</u>.

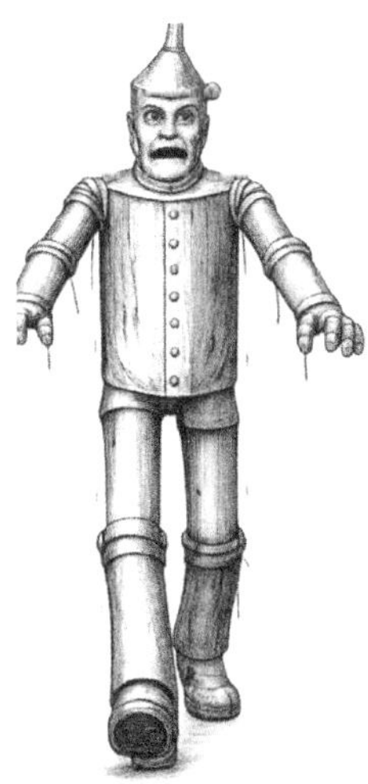

The Weight–Pain–Inflammation Loop

- Inflammation rises.
- Insulin signaling becomes disrupted.
- Cravings intensify.
- Weight sticks.
- Joints ache.
- Movement decreases.
- Inflammation increases again.

It's not in your head — it's your biology responding.

At this stage, you don't need to understand insulin in detail. What matters is recognizing that **poor metabolic signaling and chronic inflammation feed off each other**.

Lowering inflammation removes friction from your metabolism and sets the stage for everything that follows.

Chapter 5:
Move Like You Mean It (Even If Your Knees Disagree)

Movement after 50 isn't about punishment or proving anything. It's lubrication. It keeps your joints, muscles, and metabolism functioning smoothly.

Maria, 70 — A Real-World Win

Maria started with a humble 5-minute walk. By the end of the 90-day plan, she comfortably walked 20 minutes and even *looked forward* to it.

Why Movement Matters

- Improves circulation
- Reduces inflammation
- Increases mobility
- Boosts mood
- Supports fasting
- Improves longevity

Joint-Friendly Movement Ideas

- Water aerobics
- Stretching
- Gentle yoga
- Resistance bands
- Chair exercises
- Slow walks

Try This Today: The 20-Step Rule

After every seated period longer than 45 minutes, get up and take 20 steps or any movement activity — anywhere, anyhow. It keeps your joints from stiffening like cold glue.

Chapter 6:
The Long History of Not Eating—On Purpose

(Why fasting is normal, human, and older than breakfast)

If you have felt like intermittent fasting feels new, trendy, or a little suspicious, you're not alone. It sounds like something invented by influencers with too much free time.

But fasting isn't new. It's ancient. And for most of human history, it wasn't optional.

Before Grocery Stores, There Was Survival

For early humans, eating followed a simple pattern: sometimes food was available, and sometimes it wasn't.

There were no refrigerators, no drive thrus, and definitely no alarms telling you it was time for a snack.

Hunters didn't wake up, eat breakfast, hunt lunch, and grab a protein bar mid-afternoon. If the hunt didn't go well, they didn't panic — they adapted.

And here's the important part:

They didn't get weak. They didn't get foggy. They didn't collapse because they "missed breakfast."

When food wasn't available, the human body flipped a metabolic switch. Stored fat was released. Ketones were produced. Energy increased. Focus sharpened. The hunting and foraging succeeded. They feasted and their bodies were refueled.

Fasting wasn't a threat — it was a survival advantage.

Why Early Humans Didn't Fall Apart Without Constant Food

When food wasn't available, the human body didn't panic — it adapted.

This wasn't because our ancestors were tougher or more disciplined. It was because the human metabolism is designed to switch fuel sources when needed.

That ability — called metabolic flexibility — helped humans survive long before modern food systems existed.

What matters here is that you understand this:

Your body was never meant to rely on constant eating to function well.

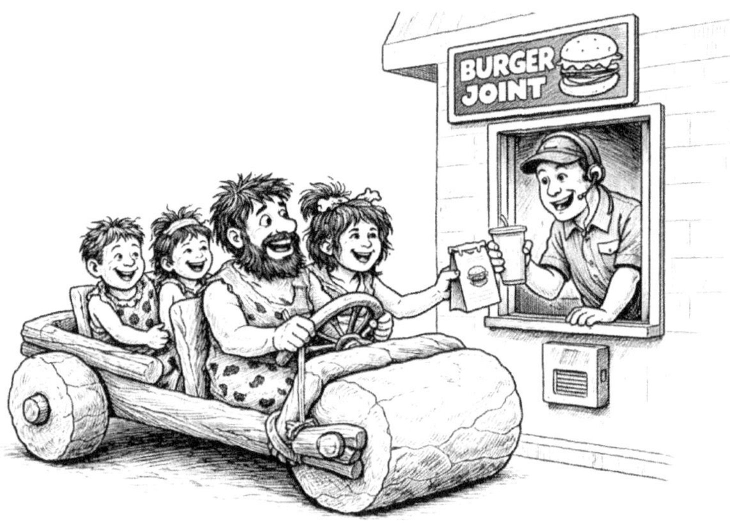

Ancient Thinkers Understood the Power of Fasting

Long before nutrition labels and calorie charts, ancient philosophers noticed something interesting.

Periods of fasting seemed to sharpen the mind.

Hippocrates, often called the father of modern medicine, believed that overeating fed illness. Plato and Aristotle spoke about restraint and clarity. The Stoics viewed fasting as a way to strengthen discipline and focus.

They weren't chasing weight loss. They were chasing clarity, resilience, and self control.

And they noticed that constant eating dulled all three.

Fasting Across Cultures and Religions

Fasting also appears across nearly every major religion – not as punishment, but as reflection, discipline, and renewal.

- Christianity observes fasting during Lent.
- Islam practices daily fasting during Ramadan.
- Judaism includes fasting on Yom Kippur.
- Buddhism and Hindu traditions incorporate fasting as spiritual practice.

Different beliefs. Different reasons.

Same observation:

When food pauses, awareness increases.

The human experience consistently recognized that not eating for a time could be beneficial – mentally, physically, and spiritually.

Doctors Once Prescribed Fasting

Before modern pharmaceuticals, fasting was commonly used by physicians as part of treatment for various conditions.

It gave digestion a rest. It reduced inflammation. It allowed the body to redirect energy toward repair.

Even in the early 20th century, fasting was used clinically – particularly for metabolic and neurological conditions.

This wasn't fringe medicine. It was practical observation.

So, What Changed?

The biggest shift didn't come from biology.

It came from industry.

As societies industrialized, work schedules changed. Factory shifts demanded predictable mealtimes. Breakfast became fuel for labor. Lunch kept production moving. Dinner closed the day.

Three meals a day wasn't designed around human metabolism – it was designed around the clock.

Later, food manufacturing took things further.

Snacks were invented. Eating "every 2–3 hours" was promoted. Hunger was framed as something dangerous.

The message slowly became:

If you're hungry, something is wrong. You must eat something now.

But hunger isn't an emergency.

It's a signal that your body is sending automatically due to the non-stop eating.

Constant Eating Is the Real Experiment

From a historical perspective, constant eating is the new behavior – not fasting.

Our ancestors fasted by circumstance. Philosophers fasted for mental clarity. Religions fasted for clarity and by tradition. Doctors prescribed fasting to treat conditions and diseases.

Modern humans snack by habit.

Fasting isn't rebellion. It isn't deprivation. It isn't extreme.

It's a return to a metabolic rhythm your body recognizes.

Why This Matters

As we age, metabolism becomes less forgiving. Insulin stays higher. Inflammation lingers. Recovery slows.

Fasting restores something that time eroded – metabolic flexibility.

It reminds your body how to switch fuel sources. It lowers insulin naturally. It supports cellular repair.

And it does so without force.

A Calm Reframe

Intermittent fasting isn't about pushing. It's about allowing.

Allowing insulin to fall. Allowing stored energy to be used. Allowing your body to do what it already knows how to do.

You're not skipping meals.

You're giving your metabolism room to work.

That makes everything that follows—ketosis, fat loss, reduced inflammation, and steadier energy—much more understandable.

Chapter 7:
Ketosis, Ketones, and Autophagy (In Plain English)

(What's happening inside your body – and why it matters)

If you've heard words like ketosis, ketones, or autophagy and felt like you needed a science degree to keep reading, relax. You don't.

This chapter is here to explain what your body is doing – no lab coat required.

What Is Ketosis?

Ketosis is not a diet. It's a metabolic state.

It simply means your body is burning fat for fuel instead of relying mostly on sugar.

Normally, when you eat carbohydrates, your body turns them into glucose. Glucose raises insulin. Insulin tells your body to store fat and burn sugar first.

When carbs are low – or when you haven't eaten for a while – insulin drops. That's the signal your body has been waiting for.

With insulin low, your liver begins converting stored fat into ketones.

That's ketosis.

What Are Ketones?

Ketones are fuel.

Clean fuel.

They're made from fat and used by your muscles, organs, and especially your brain.

Many people notice that when ketones rise:

- hunger quiets down
- energy increases
- thinking becomes clearer
- crashes disappear

That's because ketones don't spike and crash like sugar does.

They burn slowly and predictably — which is exactly what your body prefers

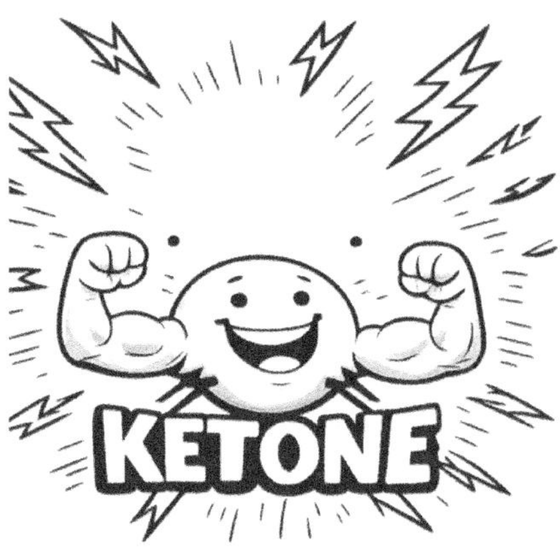

Why Ketosis Matters

As we age, insulin tends to stay higher for longer. Muscle mass decreases. Inflammation increases. And your ability to switch between fuel sources – called metabolic flexibility – weakens.

Ketosis restores that flexibility.

It reminds your body how to:

- access stored fat
- lower insulin naturally
- stabilize energy
- reduce inflammation

This isn't forcing anything.

It's reactivating a system that's always been there.

What Is the Keto Diet, really?

The ketogenic diet is simply a way of eating that supports ketosis.

It does this by:

- lowering carbohydrates
- prioritizing protein
- incorporating healthy fats

Despite what the internet might suggest, keto is not about eating sticks of butter or avoiding vegetables.

A real keto plate looks like:

- meat, poultry, or fish
- low-carb vegetables

- healthy fats like olive oil, butter, or avocado

Keto makes fasting easier. Fasting makes ketosis deeper.

They support each other.

Which Diets Fall Under the Ketosis Umbrella?

Several approaches can lead to ketosis:

- **Ketogenic diet** (low carb, moderate protein and fat)
- **Low-Carb diet** (not always ketogenic, but often close)
- **Carnivore or Ketovore** (very low carb, high nutrient density)
- **Intermittent Fasting** (works even with moderate carbs)

The common thread isn't the food label.

It's lowering insulin.

What Is Autophagy?

Autophagy is your body's built-in cleanup and recycling system.

Think of it as cellular spring cleaning.

Old, damaged proteins get broken down and reused. Cells function better. Inflammation drops.

Autophagy increases when insulin is low — especially during fasting.

This is why fasting is often linked to:

- improved cellular health
- reduced inflammation
- better aging effects

You don't need long fasts to benefit.

Even modest fasting windows can support autophagy.

A Simple Way to Think About It All

- Ketosis = burning fat for fuel
- Ketones = the fuel made from fat
- Keto Diet = eating in a way that supports ketosis
- Fasting = lowering insulin long enough for ketosis and autophagy to take effect
- Autophagy = cellular cleanup and repair

No mystery. No magic.

Just biology doing what it was always designed to do.

Why This Chapter Comes Before the Plan

Before you fast. Before you change your meals. Before you follow a schedule.

It is important for you to understand why this works.

Once you do, the next chapters stop feeling intimidating – and start feeling reasonable.

Chapter 8: The Low-Carb Sidekick That Crushes Inflammation

Keto isn't an all-you-can-eat bacon contest. It's a simple, inflammation-focused way of eating built around protein, healthy fats, and low-carb veggies.

NOTE: It's important to emphasize that the keto diet isn't mandatory to successfully practice intermittent fasting. Fasting alone is effective, but I can't stress enough how much the keto diet simplifies the process. Why? When someone consumes high-carbohydrate foods, they often experience more intense hunger and cravings during fasting, making it difficult to maintain. I recommend starting with keto and intermittent fasting together. Once you're keto-adapted, you can decide if you want to continue. If keto isn't for you, there's still plenty of valuable information in this book to guide you through your intermittent fasting journey. You also have the option to skip the keto diet content and jump right into intermittent fasting.

Carlos, 60, was skeptical

He thought keto meant eating butter straight from the stick. Then he learned keto meals included steak, chicken, salmon, soups, and avocado bowls. His shoulders relaxed. "Oh," he said. "I can do that."

Why keto works better as we age

- lowers inflammation
- reduces cravings
- stabilizes blood sugar
- improves mental clarity
- keeps hunger under control

Keto prepares your body. ***Fasting*** accelerates it.

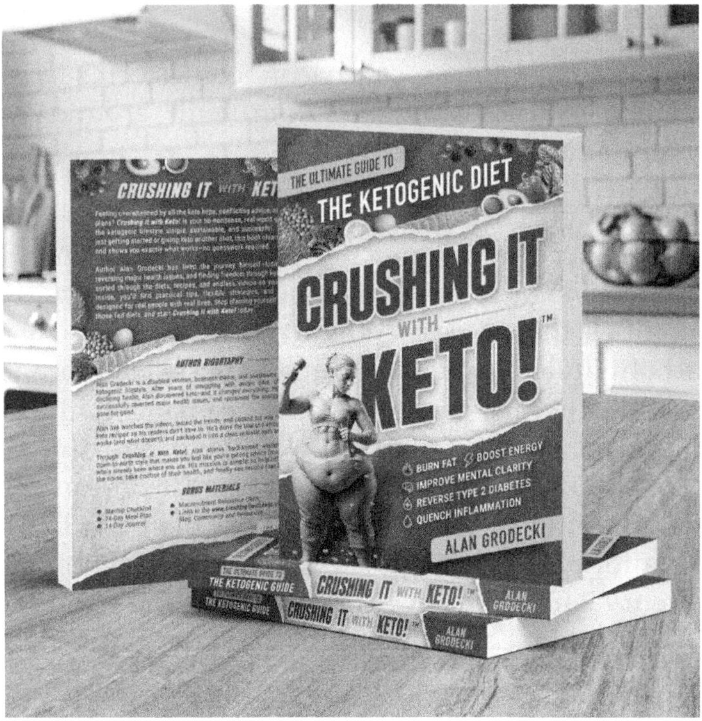

If you are interested in learning more about the ketogenic diet, I published a useful guide. You can order it on Amazon with this link - https://bit.ly/4lyRYvy or simply scan the QR Code below using the camera on your phone.

Chapter 9:
Keto + IF: The Dynamic Duo

Some things just work better together – sunshine and weekends, laughter and friends, keto and intermittent fasting.

Why the synergy works

- Keto keeps hunger calm.
- Fasting lowers insulin.
- Together they support steady fat loss.
- Inflammation drops.
- Energy rises.
- Cravings fade.

This combo is your metabolic superpower.

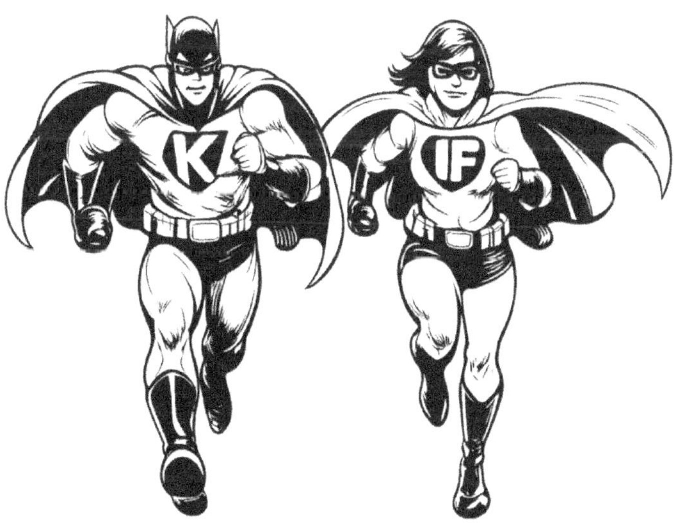

Tony, 52, noticed fast results

Keto made fasting easier. Fasting made keto stronger. His belly fat finally surrendered.

Safety First: We're Getting Healthy, Not Trying to Break Olympic Records

Before we go any further, let's slow things down and talk safety.

Fasting should always be:

- gradual
- hydrated
- flexible
- adjusted to your body

If you take medication, talk with your healthcare provider before changing your eating schedule.

Electrolytes (sugar-free) matter. Hydration matters. And if something feels wrong – stop.

Progress comes from consistency, not pushing.

Your health always comes first.

Chapter 10:
How to Read a Nutrition Label Without Needing a PhD

(Finding sugars, carbs, and sneaky oils hiding in plain sight)

One of the fastest ways to stall progress – even when you're eating "healthy" – is getting fooled by the food labels.

This chapter isn't about turning you into a nutrition detective or making grocery shopping miserable. It's about giving you a few simple skills so you can spot problems quickly and move on with your life.

If you can read a nutrition label with confidence, keto and intermittent fasting become dramatically easier.

For more details, here the web address for the FDA website - https://www.fda.gov/food/nutrition-food-labeling-and-critical-foods

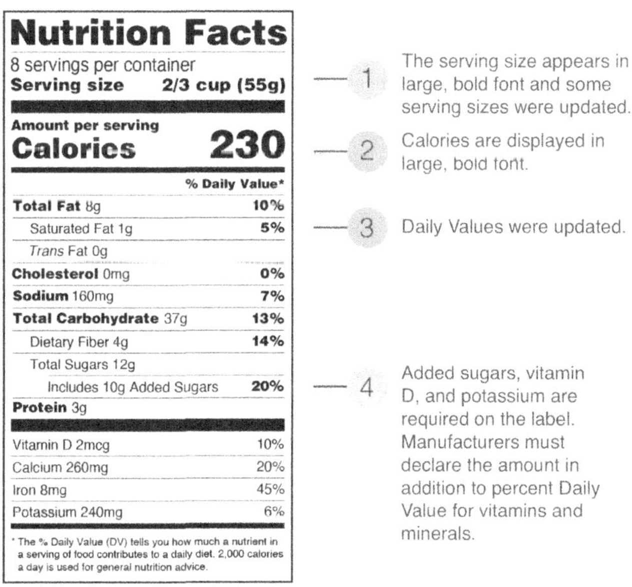

Why Labels Matter

As you age, your margin for error gets smaller. Foods that once caused only mild bloating or fatigue can now trigger:

- joint pain
- inflammation
- cravings
- energy crashes
- stubborn weight stalls

The problem isn't willpower.

It's often hidden ingredients quietly spiking insulin and inflammation.

Start With the Ingredient List (Not the Big Numbers)

The ingredient list tells the truth.

Manufacturers can make the front of a package say almost anything. The ingredient list is regulated — and listed in order of quantity. Pay attention to the ingredients listed first on the label.

If sugar or refined grains appear in the first few ingredients, that food will work against your goals.

The Many Names for Sugar

Sugar rarely shows up as just "sugar."

Watch for:

- cane sugar
- corn syrup

- high-fructose corn syrup
- rice syrup
- maltodextrin
- dextrose
- fructose
- evaporated cane juice
- honey or agave (still sugar)

If you see several forms of sugar sprinkled throughout the list, that's intentional. If an ingredient ends with "-ose", it is sugar. If it ends with "-ol" it may be a sneaky sugar alcohol.

Understanding Carbohydrates Without Obsessing

Macronutrients (Macros) consist of carbohydrates, fat and protein. By the way - Sugar is a carbohydrate. On the nutrition label, you'll see:

- Fat
- Carbohydrate
- Protein

For keto and fasting success:

- total carbs matter
- fiber doesn't spike insulin
- sugars <u>always</u> spike insulin

You don't need to count every gram — just notice patterns.

Foods with high carbs and low fiber rarely support your goals.

Net Carbs: Helpful, But Not Magic

Net carbs are calculated by subtracting fiber from total carbohydrates.

This can be useful — but it's not a free pass.

Highly processed "keto" foods can technically be low net-carb while still:

- spiking insulin
- triggering cravings
- stalling progress

Whole foods beat the math every time. Try to avoid manufactured or processed foods.

The Oil Problem (Quiet but Powerful)

Industrial seed oils are one of the biggest drivers of modern inflammation. These are literally engineered oils that have been highly processed and in many cases are hydrogenated to prevent them from becoming rancid.

Watch for:

- soybean oil
- canola oil
- corn oil
- sunflower oil
- safflower oil
- grapeseed oil

These oils are inexpensive, shelf-stable, and heavily used — but they are not friendly to metabolic health. You will commonly find these oils listed as the first ingredient in salad dressings, mayonnaise, and many other dressings and sauces.

Better options include:

- olive oil
- avocado oil
- butter

- ghee
- coconut oil
- lard
- tallow

There are keto-friendly products widely available. You don't need perfection – just awareness.

Serving Sizes: The Optical Illusion

Serving sizes on the label are often unrealistically small.

A "serving" might be:

- half a bar
- a few chips
- a spoonful smaller than you'd ever eat

Always glance at:

- servings per container

That single bag or bottle is often two to four servings, whether the label admits it or not. If the label uses smaller portions, they can make the nutrition numbers look better to the average consumer (intentional or not).

Nothing sucks worse than finishing a snack, then flipping over the package to find out you just ate 8 servings. Look before you leap.

Marketing Words That Mean Very Little

These phrases sound comforting but aren't regulated:

- natural
- wholesome

- heart-healthy
- low-fat (usually means high sugar)
- made with whole grains

They don't guarantee low sugar, low carbs, or low inflammation. The newest angle is pushing "high protein" on the label as a feel-good distraction from the "real" ingredients.

Flip the package over.

A Simple Label-Reading Checklist

Ask yourself:

- How many servings are in the package?
- What are the first ingredients?
- Do I recognize most of the ingredients?
- Are sugars listed early?
- What about added sugars?
- Are seed oils present?
- Is the carb load reasonable?
- Would this food keep me satiated (satisfied)?

If the answer feels shaky, put it back.

There's no drama in choosing something else.

The Big Picture

Nutrition labels aren't there to scare you.

They're there to give you clarity.

Once you know what to look for, shopping gets easier – not harder.

And when food stops quietly working against you, keto and fasting become easier, cravings calm down, and inflammation drops naturally.

That's not just label discipline.

That's alignment.

Chapter 11: Dining Out Without Blowing It

(How to stay keto-friendly at restaurants, parties, and social events)

One of the biggest worries people have when starting keto and/or intermittent fasting isn't hunger – it's real life.

Birthdays happen. Friends invite you out. Restaurants exist. And unless you plan on living alone with a slow cooker forever, you need a way to navigate social eating without stress or regret.

The good news? Eating out doesn't ruin progress.

Not knowing how to eat out does.

First, Let's Lower the Pressure

You are not on a diet.

You are building a lifestyle.

That means flexibility matters more than perfection. One meal does not undo progress – especially when insulin and inflammation are already under control.

The goal when eating out isn't to be flawless.

It's to be intentional.

The Simple Restaurant Rule

When in doubt, ask yourself one question:

"What would this meal look like if carbs weren't the star of the plate?"

Then build from there.

Most restaurants already serve keto-friendly meals – they're just buried under bread, fries, or sugary sauces.

You can usually find keto-friendly options offered on the menu.

Easy Keto Wins at Almost Any Restaurant

You can almost always choose:

- steak or grilled meat
- chicken or fish
- eggs or omelets
- burgers without the bun
- salads with protein (skip the sugary dressings and croutons)
- vegetables sautéed in butter or olive oil

Don't be shy about substitutions. Restaurants expect them.

I have dined out enough times that I always have an idea what works. Pro Tip - Look at the restaurant menu on your device before you go. That way, you are more confident and there is no longer that pressure to decide on the spot.

What to Watch Out For

The biggest keto traps when eating out aren't desserts – they're the sauces and sides.

Be cautious with:

- salad dressings
- sweet glazes
- marinades
- barbecue sauce

- honey mustard
- teriyaki
- breaded coatings

A simple question solves most of this:

"Can I get that without the sauce?"

Fast Food Without the Fallout

Sometimes convenience wins.

You can still stay on course:

- burger patties without buns
- grilled chicken sandwiches without bread
- breakfast bowls without hash browns
- eggs, sausage, bacon
- Chef salad without the croutons (essentially a hardy sandwich without the bread)

It's not gourmet — but it works.

Social Events, Parties, and Buffets

Scan first.

Look for:

- meat
- cheese
- vegetables
- eggs
- salads

Eat those first and you may find that you are satisfied.

If you want a small indulgence afterward, decide consciously – not impulsively.

Alcohol: Let's Be Honest

Alcohol hits harder on keto and fasting.

If you choose to drink:

- stick to dry wine
- choose spirits with soda water
- avoid sugary mixers
- eat protein first

If you feel you need to have a drink in your hand to be social; order a mocktail (I prefer club soda with a lime). Bartenders are usually keen to the needs of their patrons.

And remember – alcohol immediately stops ketosis and pauses fat burning.

That's useful information, not judgment.

When You Do Go Off-Plan

It will happen.

The mistake isn't the meal – it's what people do after the meal.

Don't punish yourself. Don't quit.

Just return to:

- hydration
- sugar-free electrolytes
- your normal fasting window
- your next keto-friendly meal

That's it.

Progress resumes immediately.

A Reframe That Changes Everything

Eating out isn't a test. It's practice.

Every restaurant meal teaches you how to make better choices next time – without stress or fear.

When you know how to maneuver real life, keto and fasting stop feeling fragile. They become sustainable.

Chapter 12:
Cravings, Stress & That 9 PM Kitchen Ambush

Cravings are not a moral failure. They're misfiring hunger hormones paired with emotion.

Stress, boredom, loneliness, frustration – they all whisper: "Let's go to the kitchen."

Enter Tony (Again)

Tony wasn't eating because he was hungry. He was eating because at 9:00 PM he was bored.

When he learned to recognize what was triggering his hunger signals, everything changed.

Why Cravings Happen

- insulin dips
- cortisol spikes
- boredom
- habit loops
- emotional triggers

Try This Today: The 10-Minute Rule

When cravings hit, drink water, coffee or tea (unsweetened) and wait 10 minutes. Distract yourself.

- If the craving fades → it wasn't real hunger.
- If it persists → eat something keto-friendly and simple.

Snack Ideas that limit insulin response

- boiled eggs
- handful of nuts (this is my kryptonite - limit the quantity)
- olives
- real cheese stick
- chicken slices

Chapter 13: The Different Ways to Fast

(From gentle daily fasts to longer formats – without the drama)

By now, you understand why fasting works. You know it's normal, human, and rooted in biology – not a willpower contest.

The next natural question is:

"Okay... but how do people actually do this?"

The good news is there's no single "right" way to fast. There are several formats, each with a different purpose, intensity, and learning curve.

This chapter will walk you through them – calmly, clearly, and without pushing you toward anything extreme.

Time-Restricted Eating: The Foundation

Most intermittent fasting starts here.

Time-restricted eating simply means you eat within a set window each day and fast the rest of the time. No calorie counting. No complicated rules.

This is where metabolic benefits begin.

12:12 – The Gentle Starting Line

A 12:12 fast means:

- 12 hours eating

- 12 hours fasting

For example:

Finish dinner at 7 PM

Eat breakfast at 7 AM

This may sound almost too easy – and that's the point.

For many people, just **stopping late-night snacking** creates immediate benefits:

- better digestion
- calmer hunger
- improved sleep
- lower insulin overnight

If you do nothing else but 12:12, **you are already practicing intermittent fasting**. I recommend this as your starting point.

14:10 – The Sweet Spot for Many Adults

A 14:10 fast extends the fasting window slightly:

- 14 hours fasting
- 10 hours eating

This is often where people notice:

- fewer cravings
- steadier morning energy
- less joint stiffness
- easier weight loss

Your body usually adapts to this format smoothly – especially when paired with keto-style meals. This fast is usually achieved by bumping breakfast back a couple of hours.

16:8 – The Most Popular Format

This is the format most people think of when they hear "intermittent fasting."

- 16 hours fasting
- 8 hours eating

You eat your meals within an 8-hour window.

This fast is usually achieved by skipping breakfast. Now you might be thinking "But isn't breakfast the most important meal of the day?" I'm not pointing fingers; but I can think of a few industries that may want us to believe that.

Many people find 16:8 feels surprisingly natural once insulin and hunger hormones settle down.

My wife and I practice 16:8 most of the time. I will still have my black coffee in the mornings, and we will have breakfast or brunch on Sundays. Intermittent fasting is meant to be flexible, not restrictive.

That said, 16:8 is **optional** – not mandatory.

You don't unlock bonus points for longer fasts.

OMAD – One Meal a Day

OMAD means eating one larger, nutrient-dense meal per day.

Some people enjoy the simplicity. Others find it too intense.

OMAD can work occasionally, but it's not required for success and not something this book will push on you. My wife and I do practice OMAD regularly (usually during the week), but we are not obsessive about it.

Longer Fasts: A Brief, Honest Look

There are longer fasting formats that some people use:

- **Alternate-day fasting** (eating every other day)
- **36-hour fasts** (dinner to breakfast two days later)
- **Multi-day fasts**

These approaches can have powerful metabolic effects – but they also demand careful preparation, experience, and often medical supervision.

Here's a fascinating piece of trivia:

The longest medically supervised fast on record lasted 382 days. The individual survived on water, vitamins, and electrolytes under strict medical observation – and lost a significant amount of weight.

Interesting? Yes.

Necessary for health? Absolutely not.

Why Longer Isn't Better for Everyone

Especially after 50, longer fasts may:

- elevate stress hormones
- disrupt sleep
- interfere with medications
- feel unnecessarily intense

More is not always better.

Consistency beats extremes.

What This Book Focuses On (On Purpose)

This book is intentionally built around shorter fasting windows — less than 24 hours.

Why?

Because they:

- are safer for beginners
- are sustainable
- fit real life
- lower insulin effectively
- reduce inflammation
- usually don't require medical supervision

They also deliver most of the benefits most people want — without turning fasting into a full-time job.

Looking Ahead

Extended fasting is a deep topic.

It deserves its own careful discussion, clear guardrails, and individual considerations.

That's why this book focuses on the formats that help most people feel better — not the extremely long ones that influencers use to impress strangers on the internet.

Down the road, I plan to explore extended fasting in a separate book.

For now, our goal is simple:

Use gentle, repeatable fasting to support your metabolism, reduce inflammation, and feel better — consistently.

Chapter 14:
Fasting After 50: Calm, Safe, and Way Less Dramatic Than You Think

Now that you understand what ketosis is, how fasting formats work, how to spot hidden sugars and oils, and how to dine out without derailing yourself, this chapter brings everything together in a calm, practical way.

If You're Still Nervous, Read This First

You do not need to be perfect. You do not need to fast for long hours. You do not need to feel miserable.

If all you do at first is stop snacking, choose real foods, and give your body a little more time between meals, you are already succeeding. Fasting is about calm consistency — not pushing, punishing, or proving anything.

Start where you are. Go slow. Listen to your body. That's how this works.

Fasting gets a bad reputation because people picture starving, fainting, or dramatically clutching a fridge door like a soap-opera scene. But real intermittent fasting is calm, flexible, and surprisingly easy once your body understands the signals you're sending.

Because you now know how insulin, ketones, and food choices interact, fasting no longer feels mysterious or extreme — it feels logical.

The Side Benefits Nobody Mentions (But You'll Notice Immediately)

Once you start fasting, something unexpected happens – your life actually gets simpler.

Suddenly, fasting comes with perks no one puts on the brochure:

- No cooking
- No cleaning
- No eating (at least for a while)
- Saves time
- Saves money

Some people joke that fasting is the most affordable health plan they've ever tried. Fewer meals mean fewer decisions, fewer dishes, and fewer chances to overthink food.

And when food stops running your schedule, you get something back that matters just as much as lower inflammation and fat loss:

More time and mental space.

Connie, 56, tried her first 12:12 fast

Connie didn't change everything at once. She cleaned up her meals, stopped late-night snacking, and used a simple 12:12 fasting window.

At first, her stomach growled so loudly the dog left the room.

By day three, something changed – she felt steady instead of hungry. Her energy rose. Her mind cleared. Her body relaxed.

Why fasting works better

Fasting works especially well at this stage of life because it gently addresses the changes that come with aging:

- Insulin rises more easily – fasting lowers it.
- Hunger hormones misfire – fasting helps recalibrate them.
- Digestion slows – fasting gives it a break.
- Energy becomes uneven – fasting increases it and smooths it out.

Combined with keto-friendly food choices and awareness of hidden sugars and oils, fasting becomes easier – not harder.

Fasting isn't extreme. It's your metabolism's quiet reset button – a concept supported by decades of research on insulin regulation, cellular repair, and metabolic flexibility.

Chapter 15:
How to Start Without Overthinking It

At this point, you understand the why. You know how keto and intermittent fasting work, why insulin matters, and why this approach is especially powerful after 50.

Now comes the part most books rush — actually starting.

This chapter is here to slow things down.

You don't need a perfect plan. You don't need willpower. You don't need to jump into long fasts or strict rules.

You need a simple on-ramp — one that lets your body adapt without stress.

First, Let's Redefine "Starting"

Most people think starting means changing everything at once.

It doesn't.

Starting simply means creating space between meals and removing the foods that inflame and confuse your metabolism. That's it.

Do only two things at first:

1. stop snacking between meals
2. shorten your eating window slightly

If you do this, you are already doing intermittent fasting.

Why Overthinking Backfires

As you get older, stress hits harder than it used to. Cortisol rises faster, recovery takes longer, and pushing too aggressively often stalls progress.

Overthinking creates pressure. Pressure raises stress. Stress raises insulin.

And elevated insulin is exactly what we're trying to avoid.

A calm start isn't just easier — it's metabolically smarter.

What a "Good Enough" Start Looks Like

Here's what success looks like when you begin:

- You eat real meals.
- You stop grazing.
- You drink more water.
- You add sugar-free electrolytes.
- You walk a little.

That's it.

No tracking apps. No perfection. No suffering.

Consistency beats intensity every time.

The Permission Most People Need to Hear

You are allowed to:

- start slow
- adjust as needed
- eat breakfast if your body wants it

- pause if something feels off

This is not a test of discipline.

It's a process of learning how your body responds.

Think in Signals, Not Rules

Instead of asking, "Am I doing this perfectly?" ask:

- Is my hunger calmer?
- Is my energy steadier?
- Are my cravings quieter?
- Do I feel less inflamed?
- Is my mind thinking clearer?

Those signals matter more than any schedule.

Why the Next Sections Work

The upcoming phases aren't challenges – they're training wheels.

Each phase:

- reduces inflammation first
- stabilizes hunger next
- builds confidence naturally
- allows your metabolism to do the heavy lifting

Nothing extreme. Nothing rushed.

Just a clear, calm path forward – starting now.

Chapter 16: Tracking Progress Without Obsessing (And Why It Makes the Next 90 Days Work Better)

Before we jump into the 90-day phases, we need to talk about something that quietly separates people who start from people who actually finish.

- It isn't discipline.
- It isn't motivation.
- And it definitely isn't suffering.

It's Awareness.

Most people think tracking is about control – counting, measuring, policing every bite like a food detective with a badge and a bad attitude. That's not what we're doing here.

In this book, tracking has one simple purpose:

To help you listen to what your body is telling you.

Because your body is constantly communicating. The problem is, most of us were never taught how to hear it.

Why Tracking Matters

After 50, progress doesn't always show up where you expect it first.

Sometimes the scale doesn't move… but: your energy steadies · your sleep improves · your joints ache less · your cravings calm down · your mood lifts

If you're only watching the scale, you miss the win – and

people who miss wins tend to quit.

Tracking turns invisible progress into visible momentum.

It shows you that something is happening, even before your jeans catch up.

Tracking Is Feedback, Not Judgment

Let's get something straight:

Tracking is not about being good or bad. It's not a report card. It's not a test. It's simply feedback.

When you track, you start noticing patterns: When I sleep better, fasting feels easier. · When I'm stressed, cravings show up at night. · When I eat enough protein, hunger stays quiet. · When I skip electrolytes, I feel flat.

That's not failure.

That's information.

And information is power.

What's Worth Tracking (And Why It Helps)

You don't need to track everything — just the things that tell the clearest story.

Fasting

Track the fasting window you used and how it felt. Easy? Neutral? Hard? Over time, this shows you what works for you.

Sleep

Hours slept and sleep quality matter more than most people realize. Poor sleep raises hunger and insulin – tracking helps you connect those dots.

Hunger

Was it real hunger or habit hunger? What time did it show up? Hunger patterns calm down long before weight drops.

Cravings

Cravings are messengers. Tracking them helps you spot stress, boredom, or emotional triggers – especially the famous 9 PM kitchen ambush.

Energy

Morning, afternoon, evening. Stable energy is one of the earliest signs your metabolism is improving.

Mood

Calmer, less irritable, more patient? That's not random – it's biology responding.

Movement

What you did – not how hard you punished yourself. Consistency beats intensity every time.

Macros (Lightly)

You're not micromanaging numbers. You're noticing patterns: enough protein, reasonable carbs, fats doing their job.

Victories

Non scale wins matter. Looser clothes. Clearer thinking. Saying no without feeling deprived.

Challenges

Travel, stress, social events. Writing them down keeps one tough day from becoming a quitting story.

Listening to Your Body Is a Skill (And Skills Improve with Practice)

Most of us spent decades overriding body signals.

- Eat because it's "time."
- Snack because it's there.
- Ignore fatigue.
- Push through stress.

Tracking reverses that.

It teaches you to ask:

- How did my body respond?
- What made this easier?
- What made it harder?

That's not obsession.

That's partnership.

And when you work with your body instead of against it, progress stops feeling like a fight.

Why Tracking Supercharges the 90 Day Plan

The next 90 days aren't about white-knuckling your way through a program.

They're about learning your body's patterns.

Tracking does three powerful things during the 90-day plan:

1. It shows progress before the scale moves.
2. It helps you adjust calmly instead of quitting.
3. It builds confidence – because you can see what's working.

By the end of 90 days, people who track don't just feel better – they understand <u>why</u> they feel better.

Order Your Companion Journal Today!

Simply scan the QR code with the camera on your phone or visit:

www.crushingitwithketo.com

SCAN ME

Chapter 17:
Phase 1: The Calm Before the Fat-Burning Storm (Days 1-14)

Think of this phase as your body learning to trust you again. Nothing extreme happens here — just calm, steady signals that it's finally safe to let inflammation drop and energy stabilize.

Your First-Week Checklist (Bookmark This Page)

Use this checklist during your first 7 days. You don't need to do everything perfectly — just aim to check most of these boxes most days.

☐ Drink water consistently throughout the day

☐ Add sugar-free electrolytes or salt your food generously

☐ Eat protein with every meal

☐ Remove sugar and refined grains

☐ Stop snacking between meals

☐ Begin with a 12:12 fasting window

☐ Take a 10–15 minute walk daily (any activity with movement works)

☐ Go to bed a little earlier than usual

If you complete this checklist, you are doing intermittent fasting correctly.

Phase 1 isn't about suffering. It's about stabilizing your metabolism.

Goals

- reduce inflammation
- lower cravings
- balance hunger
- improve digestion
- increase steady energy
- overall improved health

Chapter 18:
Phase 2: Fasting Training Wheels - Smooth, Simple, Zero Drama (Days 15-45)

This is where fasting stops feeling like a strategy and starts feeling like a routine. Your body knows what to expect now – and it responds by making everything easier.

Now that your metabolism has calmed down… we begin fasting gently.

The progression continues

- Week 1: 12:12 – simple, gentle, zero stress.
- Week 2: 14:10 – your body barely notices the change.
- Week 3+: Optional 16:8 – only if your body says, "Yeah, we're good."

Mark's Unexpected Morning

Mark assumed fasting would turn him into a grumpy zombie. Instead, on day 5 of doing 14:10 schedule, he woke up at 6:30 with enough energy to clean the garage. His wife stood in the doorway, confused and slightly alarmed. "Are you… okay?" she asked.

He was more than okay – his metabolism was finally cooperating.

Why Phase 2 Works So Well

Your body is learning:

- hunger doesn't control you
- insulin doesn't need to spike constantly
- energy doesn't have to crash
- cravings don't have to run the show

You're not white-knuckling anything. You're gliding.

Try This Today: The Hunger Check-In

When hunger hits, ask yourself:

- Am I thirsty?
- Am I bored?
- Am I stressed?
- Is this real hunger or "habit hunger"?

Most people discover hunger is often just a habitual nudge, not a biological alarm. If I feel hungry, I will usually drink a glass of water or have a cup of black coffee, and the hunger feeling disappears.

Chapter 19: Phase 3: The Inflammation Reset – Goodbye Stiffness, Hello Energy (Days 45-90)

By this point, you're no longer trying to change your body — you're watching it change on its own. This phase is where the payoff becomes undeniable.

Phase 3 is where the big wins show up — the ones you feel in your bones (literally).

Your fasting window is set (14:10 or 16:8). Your inflammation is dropping. Your metabolic engine is humming. Your confidence is rising.

Lisa's Victory Moment

On day 62, Lisa realized something strange: she hadn't thought about snacking all afternoon. Not once. Not even a quick glance toward the pantry.

She paused mid-thought and whispered, "Who am I?"

Common Phase 3 Wins

- Morning stiffness fades.
- Mood stabilizes.
- Belly fat begins melting.
- Afternoon crashes disappear.
- Sleep deepens.
- Cravings lose power.
- Energy feels smoother.

Your Weekly Milestones (Snapshot)

- Week 7: Digestion improves; bloating reduces.
- Week 8: Pain levels decrease noticeably.
- Week 9: Fasting feels natural – not forced.
- Week 10: Clothes fit differently… in a good way.
- Week 11: Steady fat loss continues.
- Week 12: Confidence spikes – you're in control.
- Week 13: Inflammation stays low; energy stays high.

Try This Today: The 5-Minute Reset

When you feel stressed, pause and breathe for 5 slow minutes. It resets cortisol, which makes fasting easier and inflammation lower.

Chapter 20: Fasting Together: Couples-Friendly Strategies That Actually Work

One of the biggest myths about lifestyle change is that you have to do it alone.

In reality, having a partner involved—at any level—can make intermittent fasting easier, more sustainable, and far less stressful.

This chapter is not about forcing your spouse, partner, or significant other to fast exactly the way you do. It's about creating alignment, reducing friction, and finding simple ways to support each other—even if you're following different schedules.

Why Couples Struggle With Health Changes

Many couples run into trouble not because fasting or dietary changes are hard, but because routines are shared.

- Meals are social.
- Snacking habits are shared.
- Schedules overlap.

When one person changes and the other doesn't, tension can creep in. That tension—not hunger—is often what derails progress.

The good news is that intermittent fasting is one of the most flexible approaches for couples, because it's based on timing rather than strict food rules.

Strategy 1: Share Meals, Not Schedules

You don't need identical fasting windows to succeed together.

One partner may follow a 16:8 schedule, while the other prefers 14:10 or even a traditional three-meal pattern.

The key is agreeing on shared mealtimes.

Dinner together most nights.

Optional shared lunches on weekends.

Independent or skipped breakfasts during the week.

This approach preserves connection without forcing conformity.

Strategy 2: Normalize Fasting—Don't Make It a Big Deal

Fasting works best when it's boring.

Instead of announcing, explaining, or defending your fasting window every day, treat it like any other routine.

"I'm not eating yet" is enough.

When fasting becomes normal, resistance fades.

Strategy 3: Plan One Protein-Forward Anchor Meal

Agree on one daily or near-daily meal that works for both of you.

Protein-forward dinners—meat, fish, eggs, and vegetables—tend to satisfy both fasting and non-fasting partners.

This reduces the need for separate cooking and eliminates food-related stress.

Strategy 4: Support Without Policing

Couples struggle when support turns into surveillance.

Avoid comments like:

"Should you be eating that?"

"I thought you were fasting."

Instead, offer neutral support:

"Let me know if you want company on a walk."

"I'm proud of you for sticking with it."

Progress thrives in encouragement, not control.

Strategy 5: Respect Different Paces

One partner may see results quickly. The other may take longer.

This is normal.

Metabolism, hormones, stress, and sleep differ—even within couples.

Stay focused on trends, not comparisons.

Strategy 6: Use Fasting to Simplify Life Together

Many couples discover that fasting reduces food decisions, grocery bills, and meal prep time.

Fewer meals often mean:

- Less stress.
- Less cleanup.
- More shared free time.

That extra space can be used for walks, conversations, or simply relaxing together.

The Bottom Line for Couples

Intermittent fasting does not require both partners to do the same thing.

It requires understanding, flexibility, and a shared goal of feeling better together.

When couples approach fasting as a tool for support—not a source of conflict—it becomes one of the most relationship-friendly health strategies available.

Epilogue

You didn't pick up this book because everything was fine.

You picked it up because, somewhere deep down, you knew your body still had more to give—and that you weren't done listening to it yet.

That instinct matters.

What you've done here isn't a dramatic reset or a temporary restart. It's a continuation. A course correction. A decision to work with your body instead of fighting it. And that's something you can carry forward long after this last page.

You've learned how to notice patterns. How to pay attention to signals instead of ignoring them. How to make small, intentional choices that quietly add up. None of that expires. None of it disappears when life gets busy, stressful, or unpredictable.

There will be days when progress feels obvious—and days when it doesn't. That's normal. Change rarely announces itself in big moments. More often, it shows up in subtle ways: better energy, clearer thinking, steadier moods, or the simple confidence of knowing what works for you.

Take what fits your life right now. Leave what doesn't. Revisit what you need later. Adjust as your body changes—because it will. That's not failure. That's wisdom.

The goal was never perfection. It was never rigid rules or white-knuckle discipline. The goal is progress that lasts. Progress you can live with. Progress you can return to, again and again, without guilt or burnout.

If you ever feel stuck, remember this: you now have a framework. You have awareness. You have proof that small, consistent actions matter more than dramatic promises.

This isn't the end of the journey. It's the part where you stop starting over and begin moving forward—on your terms.

Let's keep crushing it—together.

Quick Start Checklist

Your First 7 Days

- Read the early chapters to understand why fasting and keto work together.
- Choose a starting fasting window (12:12 or 14:10).
- Pick a consistent dinner cutoff time.
- Stop snacking between meals.
- Drink water consistently throughout the day.
- Add sugar-free electrolytes or salt your food generously.
- Build meals around protein first, then add healthy fats.
- Reduce sugar, refined grains, and seed oils.
- Walk 10–15 minutes daily.
- Go to bed slightly earlier than usual.

What to Track (Lightly)

- Fasting window used (and how it felt)
- Sleep duration and quality
- Hunger (real vs habit)
- Cravings and triggers
- Energy levels (morning / afternoon / evening)
- Mood and stress
- Movement completed
- Wins (non-scale victories)
- Challenges (what you learned)

Daily Reminders

- Hunger is a signal, not an emergency.
- Calm consistency beats intensity.
- Insulin responds to frequency more than perfection.
- If something feels off, pause and adjust.
- One imperfect day does not erase progress.

90-Day Transformation Map

This 90-Day Transformation Map is your big-picture guide to what changes over time as your body adapts to the intermittent fasting and the ketogenic lifestyle. Progress is not linear, and everybody is different – but these milestones help you to recognize wins beyond the scale.

Phase 1: Stabilize & Calm (Days 1–14)

- Reduce inflammation and calm digestion
- Begin lowering insulin through reduced snacking
- Establish a gentle fasting window (12:12 or 14:10)
- Notice early hunger pattern changes
- Experience improved sleep or energy stability
- Build trust between you and your body

Phase 2: Adapt & Build Momentum (Days 15–45)

- Fasting feels more natural and less forced
- Hunger signals become quieter and more predictable
- Cravings decrease in frequency and intensity
- Energy becomes steadier throughout the day
- Optional progression to 16:8 fasting if desired
- Clothes begin fitting differently

Phase 3: Transform & Sustain (Days 46–90)

- Inflammation noticeably reduced
- Consistent fasting routine feels automatic
- Fat loss becomes more visible
- Improved mobility and joint comfort
- Sleep quality deepens
- Confidence and control increase

- Non-Scale Victories to Watch For:
    - Looser clothing
    - Clearer thinking
    - Improved mood and patience
    - Reduced joint stiffness
    - Less obsession with food
    - Greater confidence in social situations

Important Reminders

Progress does not happen all at once. Some weeks bring visible change; others build invisible foundations. Tracking your fasting, sleep, hunger, energy, and mood helps you see the full picture of transformation.

This map works best when paired with the Crushing It With Keto!™ 90-Day Journal, where daily entries turn effort into awareness and awareness into lasting change.

Order Your Companion Journal Today!

Simply scan the QR code with the camera on your phone or visit:

www.crushingitwithketo.com

SCAN ME

Thank You!

Congratulations on choosing Crushing It with Keto! ™: Intermittent Fasting Blueprint to Thrive After 50: A Simple & Safe 90-Day Plan

You've made a powerful decision to take control of your health and transform your lifestyle! I'm confident Crushing It with Keto! will equip you with everything you need to achieve outstanding results and experience using the transformative power of the intermittent fasting and ketogenic lifestyle.

If you're seeing positive changes and enjoying the journey, I would greatly appreciate it if you shared this excitement by following me on my Author Page along with leaving a 5-star review. Your feedback is incredibly valuable. Not only does it support our work, but it also helps inspire and guide others toward their own success.

Thank you for your commitment to a healthier, happier life. I have no doubt you're going to crush it!

Warmest Regards,

Alan Grodecki

Author Page

https://bit.ly/4sgoExw

Printed in Dunstable, United Kingdom

79330618R00058